EQUINE ESSENTIAL OILS

Cheryl W. Rennels

Second Printing April 2008
First Printing September 2006

Copyright © 2008 Beneficence, Inc.
Livermore, Colorado
www.beneficence.net   970-222-5184   cheryl@beneficence.net

ISBN: 0-9788394-0-4
Printed in the United States of America

Published by: *Beneficence*
Power Spirit Freedom Movement

A spirit-centered business for consciousness.
Gratitude to all who come forth to present their full potential.
Supporting all those standing in their gifts.
Allowing the freedom to move in spirit on this earth.
Your power...   Your spirit...
Your freedom...   Your movement!

Publishing ◆ Private Consulting ◆ Books ◆ Products ◆ Classes ◆ Outreach

For People ◆ For Animals

be·nef·i·cence (bə-nef′ə-sens), *n.* actively doing good.

If you talk to the animals
they will talk with you
and you will know each other.
If you do not talk to them
you will not know them,
and what you do not know
you will fear.
What one fears
one destroys.

Chief Dan George
(Geswanouth Slahoot, 1899-1981)
Chief of the Tsleil-Waututh
Writer, Oscar-nominated Actor

EQUINE ESSENTIAL OILS

Table of Contents

ACKNOWLEDGMENTS

First and foremost, I acknowledge and bless the horses. They trusted me with the situations and symptoms they brought me. Each lesson taught me something new and different. With this knowledge I could, in turn, assist another horse, human, or other species. Unlike humans, horses don't question, judge or anticipate. They accept the energy of the oils at the simplest level—the vibration or resonance.

My journey with essential oils began in 2001 when I went to a Young Living Essential Oils workshop presented by Claudia Lanigan. In her skilled hands, I learned about the power of oils and to trust the application of the oils. My husband, Duane Rennels, encouraged me to attend the workshop and stayed by my side as I used the products for the first time to augment traditional veterinary treatment.

I rely on naturopathic doctor D. Gary Young's passion to research and produce pure and powerful therapeutic-grade essential oils. His pioneering spirit in creating Young Living Essential Oils allows me, as a distributor, to avail myself of the current international research surrounding the essential oil industry. Cecelia Keenan taught me "Energy Recalibration," which led me to trust and use kinesiology as a valuable tool in my everyday life. G. W. Hardin advised and counseled me on life's spiritual path and the vastly more complicated world of publishing. Sandy Lagno walked into my life in 2006 and deepened my understanding of equines and how they view humans and complementary treatments.

My sincere gratitude goes to all my human clients and various friends and relatives who have supported me from the beginning. They trusted my advice when I asked them to learn about essential oils by using them. This journey has been about trust. Young Living Essential Oils have forever changed my life and the lives of the horses with whom I have worked.

In addition, I extend a special thanks to the team working in the background. Your help and support made this dream a reality.

Copy Editor: Carol Spiciarich Mahoney
Mahoney Consulting, LLC

Cover Design: G. W. Hardin
www.gwhardin.com

Editor: Ann Streett-Joslin
www.RanchoVistaLLC.com

DISCLAIMER

The information in this book is for educational purposes only and is complementary to traditional veterinary care. It is not intended to prevent, diagnose, prescribe, treat, or heal any condition for humans, horses, or other animals. Statements made within this book have not been evaluated by the Food and Drug Administration. Please read the <u>SAFETY GUIDELINES</u> chapter later in this book and consult with your health care professional. Young Living Essential Oils distributors may answer questions you have about the products. The author, Cheryl W. Rennels, and publisher, Beneficence, Inc., and any others involved in the creation of this book, shall have neither responsibility nor liability to any person or entity with respect to any loss or damage caused or alleged to be caused, directly or indirectly, by the information in this book.

INTRODUCTION

This book, *Equine Essential Oils,* is meant to be simple because horses are simple and straightforward. It is in simplicity of information that we find clarity in the message of this book.

Equine Essential Oils is about products and methods that are effective and synergistic to the well-being of the horse. These products and methods are entirely complementary to traditional veterinary care. The only oils referenced in this book are Young Living Essential Oils, for they are the only oils I have found to be effective. I rely on their consistent standards for purity in the vibration or resonance of each oil.

The information provided in *Equine Essential Oils* is from my personal experience and the materials listed in the REFERENCES chapter later in this book. This information is not meant to cure or heal, for those are human concepts. It is my belief that by inhaling or applying an essential oil, the individual vibration of that oil is set into action. It is through this vibration that the horse can move into harmony and, thus, into physical and emotional balance.

Prior to using this information for your horse, please read the DISCLAIMER chapter and the SAFETY GUIDELINES chapter in this book and follow them closely. Once you have done this, you will be ready to start discovering for yourself the benefits of using essential oils on horses. The horses and you are ready.

SAFETY GUIDELINES

- Treat essential oils as you would any product recommended for health care by your horse's veterinarian.

- Always consult with your horse's veterinarian.

- Keep essential oils out of the reach of children.

- Keep bottles tightly closed and out of direct sunlight, as some essential oils are photosensitive.

- Avoid excessive temperatures, as some oils are heat sensitive.

- Keep essential oils out of or away from:
  - the eyes
  - the sensitive skin around the eyes
  - the ears
  - the genitals and rectum

- Essential oils may damage contact lenses.

- Keep essential oils away from open flames and candles, as some oils may be flammable.

- Prior to internal consumption of any essential oil, see "Essential Oils Certified as GRAS or Food Additives by the FDA."[1]

---

1. *Essential Oils Desk Reference*, page 431.

WHAT IS AN ESSENTIAL OIL?

Evidence of essential oils dates back to 4500 BC. They were used for their medicinal and aromatic properties. Essential oils are derived from unique liquid plant compounds, which are the "life blood" of the plant and are vital for its growth and as a natural defense against insects and disease.

Humans and animals can benefit from essential oils in the same manner as plants. Essential oils and blood have many common properties, including constituents for regeneration and hormone-like chemicals.[2]

The human body readily identifies and accepts essential oils because of similarities in the chemical structure of plants and human cells. In order for the chemical content to work best with the body, the plant's environment when grown and distilled must be of the highest standards.

Young Living Essential Oils do not sit on the skin and are not greasy. They easily penetrate the skin due to their lipid-soluble structure. Horses generally respond to essential oils in much the same way as humans. Refer to the <u>LESS IS MORE: HOW TO USE ESSENTIAL OILS WITH EQUINES</u> chapter later in this book.

---

2. *Essential Oils Desk Reference*, page 8.

THERAPEUTIC-GRADE ESSENTIAL OILS

> Young Living offers pure, unadulterated essential oils, essential oil blends, and oil-enhanced products. At Young Living, in-house and independent laboratory testing shows that [their] essential oils meet high industry standards that qualify them as "therapeutic grade." This means that health professionals choose them for promoting health and wellness.[3]

This is my reason for using Young Living products for horses and myself. The company's distillation process retains as many chemical compounds from the plant as possible. The climate, soil conditions, and harvesting methods are considered prior to plant selection. Plants selected for distillation are free from chemicals and other toxic compounds, and the distillation process is of the highest standards.

Each essential oil has a unique chemical signature that is identified through a chemical profile. The purity of each oil gives it its unique therapeutic properties and aroma.

The use of inferior oils, such as synthetic or adulterated oils, will not produce the therapeutic properties desired. Young Living Essential Oils are graded according to the Association French Normalization Organization Regulation (AFNOR) and International Standards Organization (ISO) standards.[4] These organizations set the standards for therapeutic-grade essential oils as compared to lower-grade oils with a similar aroma.

---

3. *Essential Oils User's Guide*, page 2.
4. *Essential Oils Desk Reference*, page 7.

LESS IS MORE: HOW TO USE ESSENTIAL OILS WITH EQUINES

<u>Minimalist Approach</u>

Equine Essential Oils is written about, and in cooperation with, horses. Sandy Lagno, interspecies translator and author of *Horses: From Our Side of the Fence*, translates this message from the horses about the use of essential oils with their species. This is what the horses want you, the reader, to know!

> *Humans - hear us*
>
> *Vibration liquids* [essential oils] *resonate powerfully on our bodies*
>
> *Humans - ask us* [before] *placing vibration liquid upon our bodies*
>
> *We ask humans - respect horse wisdom of knowing*
>
> *We ask humans - use vibration liquid respectfully*

There is one fundamental concept to remember when working with essential oils and horses: **Less is more!** As humans, we assume the size of the horse determines the amount of a product to use. This is not true for the horse! Equine systems are very sensitive and are easily overloaded. They are very attuned to alternative or complementary products and techniques. Horses easily feel the vibration or resonance. Both externally and internally, they will tend to require fewer oils in smaller quantities than humans.

If a horse becomes overloaded with an essential oil or any other alternative/natural therapy, the intended repairing or balancing stops. The horse will actually feel discomfort. Be observant of symptoms resulting from releases or shifts within its system. The horse may have been holding on to many dysfunctional patterns that began releasing due to the vibration of the oil. Always consult with a professional when appropriate. Remember, less is more, whether the method is topical, internal, or by inhalation.

The Process

Using essential oils is an ongoing commitment to the well-being of your horse. It takes time, sometimes many months, for a horse to move through the many layers of an issue, whether physical or emotional. Each horse resonates differently to the oils, therefore, the process of moving into balance will be different for each horse.

Over time, different oils will be needed on different areas or with different techniques. In fact, if your horse requires the same oil in the same location day after day, then movement is not occurring. If this is the case, look for another technique or product to use in addition to the oils. Horses and people are similar in that we are about movement, which is ongoing and will ultimately bring the horse into a balanced state of well-being.

Essential oils can be used as a treatment for a known problem or as a preventative measure. Check in with your horse from time to time or when a stressful event, such as a vet call, an injury, or a particularly strenuous ride, occurs.

Selecting Oils

The author uses various methods of kinesiology, also referred to as muscle testing or dowsing, to determine:

- when the horse can benefit from an essential oil
- which essential oil to select
- where to apply the oil
- how to administer the oil

See the <u>REFERENCES</u> chapter later in this book for resources on kinesiology.

Equine Essential Oils is meant as a guide for choosing and using essential oils for your horse. Each oil's information has two basic components listed: the physical and the spirit. The horse may choose an oil for the physical property, or its powerful spirit may desire the energetic imprint of the oil. It is important to be aware and respect the horse. Take your time to sense and observe the horse as you are approaching it with the oils. Allow the horse to smell the oils, and it will be drawn to the one it needs. Maintain a secure distance from the horse, as it may tend to reach out with its mouth and grasp that particular oil.

Applying Oils

There are three basic ways to administer essential oils with equines: topical application, internal consumption, and inhalation.

1. Topical Application

Drop the oils directly from the bottle onto the skin or hair. If dropping the oil is awkward, or if you are working around the horse's eyes or ears, first drop the oil onto your fingertips, then gently apply to the horse. Avoid contact with sensitive skin near the nose, eyes, rectum, or genital area. Keep the oils out of the eyes and ears. If application near the ear is desired, apply the oil on the hair outside of the ear. If the skin shows signs of irritation, bumps, swelling, or loss of hair, this is usually the result of a release through the skin. An application of pure vegetable oil or emu oil over the essential oil location may lessen the symptom. If your horse is prone to this skin reaction, a dilution of the essential oil in a pure vegetable oil before application may lessen the potential for a future symptom.

Key areas of application are:

- Spine: withers to dock
- Hoof: coronet band and frog
- Forehead
- Poll
- Behind and around the ears
- Shoulders
- Over vital organs

2. Internal Consumption

Essential oils that are Generally Regarded As Safe (GRAS) or certified as Food Additives (FA) by the FDA as safe for human consumption,[5] are, in my opinion, also safe for internal consumption by horses. The oils may be added to any cold or room-temperature food or liquid to be consumed. Some horses will actually lick the oil off your hand, if offered. Use caution to avoid being bitten. Refer to the <u>SAFETY GUIDELINES</u> chapter in this book.

---

5. *Essential Oils Desk Reference*, pages 19, 431.

3. Inhalation

If inhalation is preferred, simply hold an open bottle of oil a few inches below the nostrils and allow the horse to inhale. Use caution, as the horse may reach out for the oil and take it from you. The aroma will produce an effect on the mind and the body, since any fragrance travels to the limbic system of the brain. This system is the mind's processing center for memory, emotion, and smell. Because inhalation is so powerful, an oil placed on the handler's body will also have an effect on the horse's well-being. Your horse is most certainly aware of the perfumes or other cosmetics you use.

EQUINE RAINDROP TECHNIQUE

D. Gary Young, ND, founder of Young Living Essential Oils, developed the original Raindrop Technique® (RT) for humans in the 1980s. RT involves the use of essential oils dropped onto the spine, in conjunction with unique movements of the practitioner's hands. The intent of this technique is to align the spine structurally and electrically. RT was adapted for equines by Heather Mack, VMD, and is called Equine Raindrop Therapy.

> It is not a cure-all, but it is a wonderful way to keep horses healthy and comfortable in their bodies. It is also a powerful addition to antibiotics when fighting an infection because it assists in strengthening the immune system. [Equine Raindrop Therapy] pulls viruses and toxins out of the system and balances the structural and electrical alignment of the horse.[6]

Dr. Mack's technique involves using the same specific oils in specific locations for every horse. Refer to the <u>REFERENCES</u> chapter later in this book.

With my experience and training, I have found that each horse is different in its need for the oils. I have been open to the feedback the horses have given me and have adapted various techniques to meet the needs of their systems. As a result, I have developed the Equine Balance Techniques explained in the following chapter.

---

6. Mack, *Raindrop Therapy: Raindrop Therapy is Good for You, Good for the Horse, and Good for the Industry.*

EQUINE BALANCE TECHNIQUES

The Equine Balance Techniques were developed from my experience using essential oils on horses. Each technique involves different oils in different amounts and creates a space for the horse to come into balance with its individual expression. All of the techniques involve the equine spine, for the overall well-being and balance of the equine spine is of utmost importance.

Four techniques are listed:

1. Equine Balance Blend™ Raindrop
2. Balance Stress Raindrop
3. Vaccination & Injection Raindrop
4. Immune System Raindrop

I have observed that most horses have common responses to the oils. If a horse has not been exposed to essential oils before, it may be wary or may try to take the bottle of oil out of your hand. Many horses are determined to smell each essential oil prior to its application. These are interesting responses to observe. It is important to respect the horse as another being by observing or sensing whether it wants the oils, before deciding to use them on the horse.

After applying essential oils topically, the skin may show signs of irritation, bumps, swelling, or loss of hair. This is normally the result of a release through the skin. If the horse looks uncomfortable, simply apply a thin coat of pure vegetable oil or emu oil on the location.

All of the Equine Balance Techniques follow the same protocol. Drop the oils where directed, then, simultaneously, gently touch one hand over the withers and another over the dock for approximately one minute.

After completing an Equine Balance Technique, retire the horse to a quiet, solitary location out of the sun, so that the effect of the technique may continue.

1. Equine Balance Blend™ Raindrop

Equine Balance Blend Raindrop uses a custom oil blend for *general balancing of the horse's emotional and physical systems.* As with the Equine Raindrop Therapy, the Equine Balance Blend Raindrop (EBBR) *strengthens the immune system* and allows for *general overall well-being.* Unlike some essential oil techniques, the EBBR will not overload the horse's system. Instead, it *allows a release, balance, or movement that is beneficial to each individual horse.*

Cheryl Rennels formulated Equine Balance Blend™ using a custom proportion of the Young Living Essential Oils cypress, ledum, frankincense, orange, peppermint, and ylang ylang. Once Equine Balance Blend is dropped onto the equine spine, specific properties of these oils—anti-inflammatory, circulatory stimulant, antibacterial, immunostimulant, and antispasmodic—allow for a powerful synergistic action. E-mail the author at Cheryl@eOneness.net to place an order for a bottle of Equine Balance Blend.

a. Drop Equine Balance Blend onto the equine spine in the order indicated.

   1. Atlas (behind the poll) ....3 drops
   2. On the spine above the point of the hip .... 1 drop
   3. Withers...3 drops
   4. Dock .... 1 drop

b. Simultaneously, gently touch one hand over the withers and another over the dock for approximately one minute.

c. Retire the horse to a quiet, solitary location out of the sun, so that the effect of the technique may continue.

2. Balance Stress Raindrop

To obtain overall balance prior to or following stress.

a. Drop the Young Living Essential Oils in the order indicated. For the forehead and poll, place the oils on your fingertips and gently apply them to the horse.

1. Clarity ....Forehead.............................. 1 drop

2. PanAway ....Croup.................................4 drops

3. Lavender ....Withers....................1 drop per side

4. Oregano..................Heel........................1 drop per hoof

5. Peace & Calming ....Poll .... 1 drop

6. Lavender ....Spine: withers to dock.......12 drops

b. Simultaneously, gently touch one hand over the withers and another over the dock for approximately one minute.

c. Retire the horse to a quiet, solitary location out of the sun, so that the effect of the technique may continue.

3. Vaccination & Injection Raindrop

Following vaccinations or injections.

a. Drop the Young Living Essential Oils in the order indicated. For the poll, place the oil on your fingertips and gently apply it to the horse.

1. Purification...........Poll..2 drops

2. ImmuPower..........Dock...2 drops

3. Clove....................Withers.....................2 drops per side

4. Gentle Baby ....Spine: withers to dock..........12 drops

b. Simultaneously, gently touch one hand over the withers and another over the dock for approximately one minute.

c. Retire the horse to a quiet, solitary location out of the sun, so that the effect of the technique may continue.

4. Immune System Raindrop

Strengthens the immune system.

a. Drop the Young Living Essential Oils in the order indicated. For the forehead, place the oil on your fingertips and gently apply it to the horse.

1. Joy ....Forehead........................... 1 drop

2. Melrose ....Frog......................1 drop per foot

3. Peace & Calming ....Withers.................1 drop per side

4. Gentle Baby ....Spine: withers to dock....10 drops

b. Simultaneously, gently touch one hand over the withers and another over the dock for approximately one minute.

c. Retire the horse to a quiet, solitary location out of the sun, so that the effect of the technique may continue.

OTHER USES

I often hear horse owners say, "You can't use anything on my horse that you don't first use on me." Perfect. Essential oils work much the same way with horses, humans, and canines. Refer to the <u>LESS IS MORE: HOW TO USE ESSENTIAL OILS WITH EQUINES</u> chapter in this book.

Extreme caution should be taken when using essential oils with the feline and avian species. Certain oils can cause harm or even kill cats and birds. Some of the differences can be attributed to metabolic factors and others to overall sensitivities. Consult with your animal's veterinarian or health care professional.

REFERENCES

Ordering Information:

Cheryl W. Rennels may be reached for private consultations, classes, or for ordering products at:
- E-mail: Cheryl@eOneness.net
- Web: www.eOneness.net

Young Living Essential Oils may be purchased at www.onewithoils.com.

Book References:

Essential Oils Desk Reference, 3rd Edition, Essential Science Publishing, 2006.

Essential Oils User's Guide, Young Living Essential Oils, Lehi, Utah, 2006.

Frost, Robert, *Applied Kinesiology: A Training Manual and Reference Book of Basic Principles and Practices,* North Atlantic Books, Berkeley, California, 2002.

Harding, BB, *Essential Oil Wisdom*, Beneficence, Inc., Livermore, Colorado, 2006.

Hawkins, David R., *Power vs. Force: The Hidden Determinants of Human Behavior,* Hay House, Inc., Carlsbad, California, 1995. (kinesiology)

Lagno, Sandy, *Horses: From Our Side of the Fence,* Beneficence, Inc., Livermore, Colorado, 2006.

Mack, Dr. Heather, *Equine Raindrop Therapy: Raindrop Therapy is Good for You, Good for the Horse, and Good for the Industry*, The Equine Journal, Fall #37, 2000. View at www.neweraproductions.com/Equine %20Journal.htm.

Mack, Dr. Heather, *Equine Raindrop Therapy*, New Era Productions, 2000. (video) E-mail Dr. Mack at crazyhorsedr@hotmail.com or visit www.neweraproductions.com.

Tucker, Louise (ed.), *The Visual Dictionary of the Horse,* DK Publishing, Inc., New York, 1994.

Woods, Walt, *Letter to Robin,* The Print Shoppe, Oroville, California, 2001. (kinesiology) Order at www.dowsers.org or www.lettertorobin.org.

ESSENTIAL OILS SELECTED FOR EQUINES

(Listed alphabetically)

AROMA SIEZ

Young Living Essential Oils Blend

The Physical

> ➤ Relieves tense muscles from physical or emotional stress

> ➤ Headaches

The Spirit

> ➤ Relaxes & calms when tense about a fearful event

BASIL

Ocimum basilicum
Young Living Essential Oils

The Physical

> ➤ Infections

> ➤ Headaches

> ➤ Inflammation

> ➤ Decongestant

> ➤ Intestinal upset

> ➤ Increases flow of saliva & bile

The Spirit

> ➤ Improves mental clarity when physically overwhelmed

BRAIN POWER

Young Living Essential Oils Blend

The Physical

> Improves delivery of oxygen to brain receptor sites

> Allows accurate perception of information

> Strengthens immune system

The Spirit

> Improves integration with the surroundings when there is a perception of separation

CLARITY

Young Living Essential Oils Blend

The Physical

- ➢ Improves mental alertness

- ➢ Increases ability to process information

The Spirit

- ➢ Increases willingness to accept new information while releasing old feelings of discord

CLOVE

Syzygium aromaticum
Young Living Essential Oils

The Physical

- Infections

- Discomfort

- Inflammation

- Toothache

- Strengthens immune system

- Intestinal parasites

The Spirit

- Assists in bonding with the herd when there is a fear of not belonging

CYPRESS

Cupressus sempervirens
Young Living Essential Oils

The Physical

- ➢ Circulation
- ➢ Infections
- ➢ Nerves
- ➢ Bleeding
- ➢ Fluid retention
- ➢ Liver
- ➢ Cramps
- ➢ Scar Tissue

The Spirit

- ➢ Increases feeling of security
- ➢ Allows grounding to Mother Earth when feeling deserted

DI-GIZE

Young Living Essential Oils Blend

The Physical

> Digestion

> Nausea

> Intestinal parasites

The Spirit

> Relieves stressful emotions caused by feelings of unresolved opposites in the environment

Equine Essential Oils

ENDOFLEX

Young Living Essential Oils Blend

The Physical

➤ Hormonal balance

➤ Metabolic balance

The Spirit

➤ Improves flexibility in movement

EXODUS II

Young Living Essential Oils Blend

The Physical

- Infections

- Strengthens immune system

The Spirit

- Brings courage to release patterns created by a fearful situation

GENTLE BABY

Young Living Essential Oils Blend

The Physical

- ➢ Skin irritations

- ➢ Stress

- ➢ Inflammation

The Spirit

- ➢ Soothes & comforts

- ➢ Provides 'TLC' when feeling deserted

HELICHRYSUM

Helichrysum italicum
Young Living Essential Oils

The Physical

> - Tissue regeneration

> - Blood clots

> - Chelation

> - Scar tissue

> - Improves function of the liver

> - Improves function of the nervous & circulatory systems

The Spirit

> - Brings the physical body into balance with the willing spirit of the horse

IMMUPOWER

Young Living Essential Oils Blend

The Physical

> ➤ Strengthens immune system

> ➤ Defends against infectious elements in the environment

The Spirit

> ➤ Allows awareness & acceptance of role in the herd, even when feeling out of balance

JOY

Young Living Essential Oils Blend

The Physical

> ➤ Relieves depression

The Spirit

> ➤ Assures self-love, even when in doubt or in fear of separation

JUNIPER

Juniperus osteosperma
J. scopulorum
Young Living Essential Oils

The Physical

> Detoxifies

> Kidneys

> Skin conditions

> Circulation

The Spirit

> Supports joy & peace

> Opens path to new purpose or job
when feeling disconnected

JUVAFLEX

Young Living Essential Oils Blend

The Physical

- ➤ Detoxifies

- ➤ Cleanses liver

- ➤ Cleanses lymph system

The Spirit

- ➤ Allows time to repair

LAVENDER

Lavandula angustifolia
Young Living Essential Oils

The Physical

- Skin cuts or irritations

- Bruising

- Burns

- Bites

- Inflammation

The Spirit

- Relaxes

- Calms & balances

LEMON

Citrus limon
Young Living Essential Oils

The Physical

- ➤ Infections

- ➤ Cleanses

- ➤ Strengthens immune system

- ➤ Strengthens circulation

- ➤ Skin conditions

The Spirit

- ➤ Stimulates

- ➤ Clears the mind of old memories

- ➤ Allows honest interactions to occur

LEMONGRASS

Cymbopogon flexuosus
Young Living Essential Oils

The Physical

> ➢ Digestion

> ➢ Lymph system

> ➢ Inflammation

> ➢ Fluid retention

> ➢ Connective tissue & ligaments

The Spirit

> ➢ Calms after facing a real or
> imagined flight-or-fight situation

MARJORAM

Origanum majorana
Young Living Essential Oils

The Physical

- Infections

- Blood

- Muscles

- Digestion

- Headaches

- Parasympathetic nervous system

The Spirit

- Brings awareness and balance to all the parts of the whole

MELROSE

Young Living Essential Oils Blend

The Physical

> - Skin conditions

> - Bruising

> - Infections

> - Regeneration

The Spirit

> - Allows acceptance of rhythm

OREGANO

Origanum compactum
Young Living Essential Oils

The Physical

> ➢ Infections

> ➢ Strengthens immune system

The Spirit

> ➢ Allows acceptance of the
> environment when there is grief
> at having no choice in
> abandonment from the dam,
> herd, land, or person

PANAWAY

Young Living Essential Oils Blend

The Physical

- Bruising

- Inflammation

- Headaches

- Ligament or muscle injuries

The Spirit

- Allows acceptance of a productive job

- Allows letting go of past feelings of being overrun by a situation or event

PEACE & CALMING

Young Living Essential Oils Blend

The Physical

> Reduces depression, anxiety, or stress

The Spirit

> Creates peace & trust

PEPPERMINT

Mentha piperita
Young Living Essential Oils

The Physical

> ➢ Infections

> ➢ Digestion

> ➢ Nerves

> ➢ Inflammation

> ➢ Taste & smell

> ➢ Skin conditions

The Spirit

> ➢ Allows time to calm feelings when the situation is producing mental fatigue, confusion, or depression

PURIFICATION

Young Living Essential Oils Blend

The Physical

- ➢ Purifies cuts

- ➢ Irregularities of the hoof

- ➢ Neutralizes poisons from bites & stings

The Spirit

- ➢ Clears disruptive energy

R. C.

Young Living Essential Oils Blend

The Physical

> Bone spurs

> Respiratory congestion

The Spirit

> Allows for unfolding of life when past situations have produced feelings of grief

RAVEN

Young Living Essential Oils Blend

The Physical

> Respiratory infections

The Spirit

> Gives strength to release old memories

SARA

Young Living Essential Oils Blend

The Physical

> Releases trauma around abuse

The Spirit

> Settles inappropriate behavior due to abusive situations, which shows up as discord or lack of movement

TANSY, IDAHO

Tanacetum vulgare
Young Living Essential Oils

The Physical

- Insect repellent

- Skin conditions

- Strengthens immune system

The Spirit

- Focuses on the resolution when the situation is offensive or irritating

THIEVES

Young Living Essential Oils Blend

The Physical

> Infections

> "…[demonstrated] killing power against airborne microorganisms"[7]

The Spirit

> Provides self-protection when feeling disrespected

---

7. *Essential Oils Desk Reference*, page 123.

THYME

Thymus vulgaris
Young Living Essential Oils

The Physical

- Infections
- Digestion
- Insomnia
- Respiratory system

The Spirit

- Springs back into the present moment after physical imbalance

TRAUMA LIFE

Young Living Essential Oils Blend

The Physical

> ➤ Strengthens immune system

> ➤ Releases stress & buried emotional trauma

The Spirit

> ➤ Provides trust & reliance on present feelings when past trauma has produced feelings of being overwhelmed

TSUGA

Tsuga canadensis
Young Living Essential Oils

The Physical

> - Pain

> - Joints

> - Blood purification

> - Urinary tract

The Spirit

> - Brings emotional balance to abandonment memory

VALOR

Young Living Essential Oils Blend

The Physical

> - Boosts aerobic state of cells

> - Assists body in electrical alignment & balance

The Spirit

> - Allows courage to change

WHITE ANGELICA

Young Living Essential Oils Blend

The Physical

> ➢ Increases strength & protection in the energetic fields

The Spirit

> ➢ Animal knowing

WINTERGREEN

Gaultheria procumbens
Young Living Essential Oils

The Physical

- Bones

- Inflammation

- Lung capacity

- Liver conditions

- Muscles & joints

The Spirit

- Increases sensory awareness of surroundings when separated & feeling despair & sorrow

ABOUT THE AUTHOR

Cheryl W. Rennels grew up on a Nebraska farm, riding and raising quarter horses. Her professional life as a banker and real estate developer led her to challenge and research why the traditional answers she had received for her own health issues often led to more dysfunction.

Rennels and her husband are ranchers in Colorado and raise foundation quarter horses. Rennels has learned that her horses, like herself, respond positively to natural, complementary health care. With masterful use of kinesiology as a tool, she is able to determine which products and techniques to use with her horses and other clients. Whether working in person with her equine clients or long distance with the horse's owner, the results are obvious. The horses respond with improvement in symptoms and behavior because the root cause of the problem has been identified and addressed.

Rennels' extensive training and awareness of many equine practices, products, and practitioners give her the wisdom to identify the cause of the issue, allowing for a natural path to full expression and potential. Rennels is available for consultations and clinics.

Visit www.eOneness.net or email Cheryl@eOneness.net.

WHISPER WOMAN

(Name given to the author by the horses)

Horses flow
Horses know

Whisper woman
Hands knowing
Eyes seeing
Inner ear hearing

Horses rhythm
Humans forget
Whisper woman remembers

Horses flow movement
Remembering grows
Horses show her how they are
They are rhythm movement
Inner knowing

Humans forget
Humans forget listening
Whisper woman remembers
Listening

Touching softly
Horses bodies
Whisper woman hears and knows

Horses graciously showing her
This inner way
The path unfolds

Whisper woman
Horses come - show - know

Translated from the horses by Sandy Lagno

CPSIA information can be obtained
at www.ICGtesting.com
Printed in the USA
BVOW09s1316130517

484049BV00001B/208/P

9 780978 839406